Dermatology Residency Match Selection Criteria and Programs Requirements

By

Match A Doc

and

Residency Guide

Table of Contents

Introduction

Dermatology Residency Match

Selection Criteria and Programs Requirements

This book is the must-read and the most single important piece you buy in your battle for residency. This is the **Dermatology** Residency Match Selection Criteria and programs requirements book that contains up-to-date information about all the programs in the United States for both AMGs and IMGs. Why this book is essential to match? It has been shown that applying to programs that you don't match their minimum criteria is just waste of money and time. It is very important that you apply to those programs that you meet their requirements and this why we decided to make your life easier by gathering the information you need in one book. The information was gathered from program directors, coordinators, chiefs, faculty and residents. It includes Programs names, Programs codes, States, Addresses, Phones, Faxes, Percentage of IMGs in the programs, Minimum USMLE Step 1 and Step 2 Score Requirements, Attempts on any step, CS requirement at time of application, USCE Requirements, Cut-Off time since graduation, Programs offering couple match and Visas Sponsored or accepted. We have more than 10 years experience in the match field and our book is the proof that will help you to get the highest number of interviews to increase your chances in the match journey.

Alabama

University of Alabama Medical Center Dermatology Residency Program

Specialty: Dermatology
Program name: University of Alabama Medical Center Program
Program code: 080-01-21-010
Program type: University-based
State: Alabama
Address: University of Alabama Medical Center, EFH 414,
             1720 University Blvd, Birmingham, AL 35294
Phone: (205) 934-5189
Fax: (205) 934-5766
Percentage of IMGs in the program: 8%
Minimum USMLE Step 1 Score Requirement: 240
Minimum USMLE Step 2 Score Requirement: 240

Attempts on any step: Must pass first attempt
CS required at time of application: No
USCE Requirement: Yes
Cut-Off time since graduation: Fresh graduates only
Program offers couple match: No
Visas Sponsored or accepted: J1 visa and H1b visa

Arizona

University of Arizona Dermatology Residency Program

Specialty: Dermatology
Program name: University of Arizona Program
Program code: 080-03-21-145
NRMP Code: 1015080A2
Program type: University-based
State: Arizona
Address: University of Arizona College of Medicine, Dermatology Program,
          PO Box 245024, Tucson, AZ 85724-5024
Phone: (520) 626-6024
Fax: (520) 626-6033
Percentage of IMGs in the program: 0%

Minimum USMLE Step 1 Score Requirement:
No limits set
Minimum USMLE Step 2 Score Requirement:
No limits set
Attempts on any step: No limits set
CS required at time of application: Yes
including ECFMG certificate
USCE Requirement: Yes
Cut-Off time since graduation: No limits set
Program offers couple match: Yes
Visas Sponsored or accepted: No visa

Mayo Clinic College of Medicine (Arizona) Dermatology Residency Program

Specialty: Dermatology
Program name: Mayo Clinic College of Medicine
(Arizona) Program
Program code: 080-03-21-127
NRMP Code: 3200080C0
Program type: Community-based university
affiliated hospital
State: Arizona
Address: Mayo Clinic Arizona, Department of
Dermatology,
            13400 E Shea Blvd, Scottsdale, AZ
85259
Phone: (480) 301-4898
Fax: (480) 301-9196

Percentage of IMGs in the program: 0%
Minimum USMLE Step 1 Score Requirement: 245
Minimum USMLE Step 2 Score Requirement: 245
Attempts on any step: Must pass on first attempt including CS exam
CS required at time of application: Yes including ECFMG certificate
USCE Requirement: None
Cut-Off time since graduation: 2 years
Program offers couple match: Yes
Visas Sponsored or accepted: No visa

Arkansas

University of Arkansas for Medical Sciences Dermatology Residency Program

Specialty: Dermatology
Program name: University of Arkansas for Medical Sciences Program
Program code: 080-04-21-013
NRMP Code: 1018080C0
Program type: University-based
State: Arkansas

Address: University of Arkansas for Medical Sciences, Department of Dermatology 576,
    4301 W Markham St, Little Rock, AR 72205,
Phone: (501) 525-6551
Fax: (501) 686-7264
Percentage of IMGs in the program: 0%
Minimum USMLE Step 1 Score Requirement: No limits set
Minimum USMLE Step 2 Score Requirement: No limits set
Attempts on any step: No limits set
CS required at time of application: No
USCE Requirement: None
Cut-Off time since graduation: No limits set
Program offers couple match: Yes
Visas Sponsored or accepted: J1 visa

California

University of California (San Francisco) Dermatology Residency Program

Specialty: Dermatology
Program name: University of California (San Francisco) Program
Program code: 080-05-21-019

Program type: University-based
State: California
Address: UCSF Medical Center, Department of Dermatology Rm 420,
1701 Divisadero St, San Francisco, CA 94115
Phone: (415) 353-7879
Fax: (415) 885-7476
Percentage of IMGs in the program: 0%
Minimum USMLE Step 1 Score Requirement: 220
Minimum USMLE Step 2 Score Requirement: 220
Attempts on any step: No limits set
CS required at time of application: Yes including ECFMG certificate and PTAL/Status
USCE Requirement: Yes
Cut-Off time since graduation: No limits set
Program offers couple match: Yes
Visas Sponsored or accepted: J1 visa and H1b visa

University of California (San Diego) Dermatology Residency Program

Specialty: Dermatology
Program name: University of California (San Diego) Program
Program code: 080-05-21-018
State: California

Address: UCSD Medical Center, Division of Dermatology MC 0869,
         9500 Gilman Dr, La Jolla, CA 92093-0869
Phone: (858) 822-3958
Fax: (858) 822-6985
Percentage of IMGs in the program: 0%
Minimum USMLE Step 1 Score Requirement: 225
Minimum USMLE Step 2 Score Requirement: 225
Attempts on any step: No limits set
CS required at time of application: Yes including ECFMG certificate and PTAL/Status letter
USCE Requirement: Yes
Cut-Off time since graduation: No limits set
Program offers couple match: Yes
Visas Sponsored or accepted: J1 visa

Los Angeles County-Harbor-UCLA Medical Center Dermatology Residency Program

Specialty: Dermatology
Program name: Los Angeles County-Harbor-UCLA Medical Center Program
Program code: 080-05-12-137
State: California

Address: Los Angeles County-Harbor-UCLA Medical Center Division of Dermatology Box 458,

1000 W Carson St, Torrance, CA 90509

Phone: (310) 781-1408
Fax: (310) 781-9328
Percentage of IMGs in the program: 0%
Minimum USMLE Step 1 Score Requirement: No limits set
Minimum USMLE Step 2 Score Requirement: No limits set
Attempts on any step: No limits set
CS required at time of application: No but PTAL/Status letter required
USCE Requirement: Yes
Cut-Off time since graduation: No limits set
Program offers couple match: Yes
Visas Sponsored or accepted: J1 visa

Stanford University Dermatology Residency Program

Specialty: Dermatology
Program name: Stanford University Program
Program code: 080-05-21-020
Program type: University-based
State: California

Address: Stanford Medicine Outpatient Center, Department of Dermatology Pavilion C,
　　　450 Broadway St, Redwood City, CA 94063
Phone: (650) 721-7193
Percentage of IMGs in the program: 0%
Minimum USMLE Step 1 Score Requirement: No limits set
Minimum USMLE Step 2 Score Requirement: No limits set
Attempts on any step: No limits set
CS required at time of application: No but PTAL/Status letter required
USCE Requirement: None
Cut-Off time since graduation: No limits set
Program offers couple match: Yes
Visas Sponsored or accepted: No visa

UCLA Medical Center Dermatology Residency Program

Specialty: Dermatology
Program name: UCLA Medical Center Program
Program code: 080-05-21-017
Program type: University-based
State: California
Address: UCLA Medical Center, Division of Dermatology 52-121 CHS,
　　　10833 Le Conte Ave, Los Angeles, CA 90095-1750

Phone: (310) 825-9182
Fax: (310) 825-3613
Percentage of IMGs in the program: 0%
Minimum USMLE Step 1 Score Requirement: 240
Minimum USMLE Step 2 Score Requirement: 240
Attempts on any step: Must pass on first attempt including CS exam
CS required at time of application: Yes including ECFMG certificate and PTAL/Status letter
USCE Requirement: None
Cut-Off time since graduation: No limits set
Program offers couple match: Yes
Visas Sponsored or accepted: J1 visa

Kaiser Permanente Southern California (Los Angeles) Dermatology Residency Program

Specialty: Dermatology
Program name: Kaiser Permanente Southern California (Los Angeles) Program
Program code: 080-05-12-144
State: California
Address: Kaiser Permanente Medical Care, Residency Admin & Recruitment 5th Floor,
        393 E Walnut St, Pasadena, CA 91188
Phone: (877) 574-0002

Fax: (626) 405-6581
Percentage of IMGs in the program: 0%
Minimum USMLE Step 1 Score Requirement:
No limits set
Minimum USMLE Step 2 Score Requirement:
No limits set
Attempts on any step: No limits set
CS required at time of application: No but
PTAL/Status letter required
USCE Requirement: None
Cut-Off time since graduation: 3 years
Program offers couple match: Yes
Visas Sponsored or accepted: J1 visa and H1b
visa

University of Southern California/LAC+USC Medical Center Dermatology Residency Program

Specialty: Dermatology
Program name: University of Southern California/LAC+USC Medical Center Program
Program code: 080-05-11-015
Program type: University-based
State: California
Address: USC Norris Cancer Hospital, Ezralow Tower #5301,
    1441 Eastlake Ave, Los Angeles, CA 90033
Phone: (323) 442-0084

Fax: (323) 442-0067
Percentage of IMGs in the program: 10%
Minimum USMLE Step 1 Score Requirement: No limits set
Minimum USMLE Step 2 Score Requirement: No limits set
Attempts on any step: No limits set
CS required at time of application: No but PTAL/Status letter required
USCE Requirement: None
Cut-Off time since graduation: No limits set
Program offers couple match: Yes
Visas Sponsored or accepted: J1 visa and H1b visa

Loma Linda University Dermatology Residency Program

Specialty: Dermatology
Program name: Loma Linda University Program
Program code: 080-05-21-111
Program type: University-based
State: California
Address: Loma Linda University Medical Center, Dermatology FMO Suite 2600,
        11370 Anderson St, Loma Linda, CA 92354
Phone: (909) 558-2842
Fax: (909) 558-2442
Percentage of IMGs in the program: 0%

Minimum USMLE Step 1 Score Requirement:
No limits set
Minimum USMLE Step 2 Score Requirement:
No limits set
Attempts on any step: No limits set
CS required at time of application: Yes,
including ECFMG certificate and PTAL/Status
letter
USCE Requirement: Yes
Cut-Off time since graduation: 5 years
Program offers couple match: Yes
Visas Sponsored or accepted: J1 visa and H1b
visa

University of California (Irvine) Dermatology Residency Program

Specialty: Dermatology
Program name: University of California (Irvine)
Program
Program code: 080-05-21-014
Program type: University-based
State: California
Address: UC Irvine Medical Center, Department
of Dermatology,
          C340 Medical Sciences I, Irvine, CA
92697-2400
Phone: (949) 824-4405
Fax: (949) 824-7454
Percentage of IMGs in the program: 0%

Minimum USMLE Step 1 Score Requirement: 220
Minimum USMLE Step 2 Score Requirement: 220
Attempts on any step: No limits set
CS required at time of application: Yes including ECFMG certificate and PTAL/Status letter
USCE Requirement: Yes
Cut-Off time since graduation: No limits set
Program offers couple match: No
Visas Sponsored or accepted: No visa

University of California (Davis) Health System Dermatology Residency Program

Specialty: Dermatology
Program name: University of California (Davis) Health System Program
Program code: 080-05-21-101
NRMP Code: 1046080A0, 1046080A1
Program type: University-based
State: California
Address: UC Davis School of Medicine, Department of Dermatology Suite 1400,
        3301 C St, Sacramento, CA 95816
Phone: (916) 734-6371
Fax: (916) 442-5702
Percentage of IMGs in the program: 0%

Minimum USMLE Step 1 Score Requirement: 235
Minimum USMLE Step 2 Score Requirement: 235
Attempts on any step: No limits set
CS required at time of application: Yes including ECFMG certificate and PTAL/Status letter
USCE Requirement: Yes
Cut-Off time since graduation: No limits set
Program offers couple match: No
Visas Sponsored or accepted: No visa

Colorado

University of Colorado Denver Dermatology Residency Program

Specialty: Dermatology
Program name: University of Colorado Denver Program
Program code: 080-07-21-022
Program type: University-based
State: Colorado
Address: University of Colorado Denver School of Medicine, Mail Stop F703,

1665 Aurora Ct, Aurora, CO 80045-0510
Phone: (720) 848-0597
Percentage of IMGs in the program: 0%
Minimum USMLE Step 1 Score Requirement: 210
Minimum USMLE Step 2 Score Requirement: 210
Attempts on any step: No limits set
CS required at time of application: Yes including ECFMG certificate
USCE Requirement: None
Cut-Off time since graduation: No limits set
Program offers couple match: Yes
Visas Sponsored or accepted: J1 visa and H1b visa

Connecticut

Yale-New Haven Medical Center Dermatology Residency Program

Specialty: Dermatology
Program name: Yale-New Haven Medical Center Program
Program code: 080-08-21-023
NRMP Code: 1089080A0

Program type: University-based
State: Connecticut
Address: Yale-New Haven Medical Center,
Department of Dermatology, PO Box 208059,
        333 Cedar St, New Haven, CT 06520
Phone: (203) 785-4092
Fax: (203) 785-7637
Percentage of IMGs in the program: 0%
Minimum USMLE Step 1 Score Requirement:
210
Minimum USMLE Step 2 Score Requirement:
210
Attempts on any step: No limits set
CS required at time of application: No
USCE Requirement: None
Cut-Off time since graduation: No limits set
Program offers couple match: Yes
Visas Sponsored or accepted: J1 visa

University of Connecticut Dermatology Residency Program

Specialty: Dermatology
Program name: University of Connecticut
Program
Program code: 080-08-31-138
NRMP Code: 1094080A0
Program type: University-based
State: Connecticut

Address: University of Connecticut Health Center, Department of Dermatology MC-6231, 263 Farmington Ave, Farmington, CT 06030
Phone: (860) 679-6759
Fax: (860) 679-8801
Percentage of IMGs in the program: 0%
Minimum USMLE Step 1 Score Requirement: No limits set
Minimum USMLE Step 2 Score Requirement: No limits set
Attempts on any step: Must pass on first attempt including CS exam
CS required at time of application: Yes including ECFMG certificate
USCE Requirement: None
Cut-Off time since graduation: No limits set
Program offers couple match: No
Visas Sponsored or accepted: J1 visa

District of Columbia

Washington Hospital Center Dermatology Residency Program

Specialty: Dermatology
Program name: Washington Hospital Center Program
Program code: 080-10-21-106
Program type: Community-based University affiliated hospital
State: District of Columbia
Address: Washington Hospital Center, 6A-126, 110 Irving St NW, Washington, DC 20010-2975
Phone: (202) 877-7204
Fax: (202) 877-8024
Percentage of IMGs in the program: 0%
Minimum USMLE Step 1 Score Requirement: No limits set
Minimum USMLE Step 2 Score Requirement: No limits set
Attempts on any step: No limits set
CS required at time of application: Yes
USCE Requirement: None
Cut-Off time since graduation: No limits set
Program offers couple match: Yes
Visas Sponsored or accepted: J1 visa

Howard University Dermatology Residency Program

Specialty: Dermatology
Program name: Howard University Program

Program code: 080-10-21-025
State: District of Columbia
Address: Howard University Hospital,
Department of Dermatology,
          2041 Georgia Ave NW, Washington,
DC 20060
Phone: (202) 865-6725
Fax: (202) 865-1757
Percentage of IMGs in the program: 0%
Minimum USMLE Step 1 Score Requirement:
220
Minimum USMLE Step 2 Score Requirement:
220
Attempts on any step: Two maximum attempts
on each step
CS required at time of application: Yes
including ECFMG certificate
USCE Requirement: None
Cut-Off time since graduation: 10 years
Program offers couple match: Yes
Visas Sponsored or accepted: No visa

Florida

University of South Florida Morsani Dermatology Residency Program

Specialty: Dermatology
Program name: University of South Florida Morsani Program
Program code: 080-11-21-096
Program type: University-based
State: Florida
Address: University of South Florida College of Medicine, MDC Box 79,
            12901 Bruce B Downs Blvd, Tampa, FL 33612-4742
Phone: (813) 974-3070
Fax: (813) 974-4272
Percentage of IMGs in the program: 0%
Minimum USMLE Step 1 Score Requirement: 240
Minimum USMLE Step 2 Score Requirement: 240
Attempts on any step: Must pass on first attempt
CS required at time of application: Yes including ECFMG certificate
USCE Requirement: Yes
Cut-Off time since graduation: No limits set
Program offers couple match: Yes
Visas Sponsored or accepted: J1 visa

Jackson Memorial Hospital/Jackson Health System Dermatology Residency Program

Specialty: Dermatology
Program name: Jackson Memorial Hospital/Jackson Health System Program
Program code: 080-11-21-026
State: Florida
Address: University of Miami/Jackson Memorial Hospital, Dermatology Program (R-250),
          PO Box 016250, Miami, FL 33101
Phone: (305) 243-6742
Fax: (305) 243-6191
Percentage of IMGs in the program: 10%
Minimum USMLE Step 1 Score Requirement: 220
Minimum USMLE Step 2 Score Requirement: 220
Attempts on any step: No limits set
CS required at time of application: Yes including ECFMG certificate
USCE Requirement: Yes
Cut-Off time since graduation: No limits set
Program offers couple match: Yes
Visas Sponsored or accepted: J1 visa

Mayo Clinic College of Medicine (Jacksonville) Dermatology Residency Program

Specialty: Dermatology
Program name: Mayo Clinic College of Medicine (Jacksonville) Program
Program code: 080-11-31-125
NRMP Code: 1032080C0
Program type: Community-based university affiliated hospital
State: Florida
Address: Mayo Clinic Jacksonville, Department of Dermatology,
             4500 San Pablo Rd, Jacksonville, FL 32224
Phone: (904) 953-6341
Fax: (904) 953-0430
Percentage of IMGs in the program: 0%
Minimum USMLE Step 1 Score Requirement: 220
Minimum USMLE Step 2 Score Requirement: 220
Attempts on any step: Must pass on first attempt including CS exam
CS required at time of application: No
USCE Requirement: Yes
Cut-Off time since graduation: No limits set
Program offers couple match: Yes
Visas Sponsored or accepted: J1 visa and H1b visa

University of Florida Dermatology Residency Program

Specialty: Dermatology
Program name: University of Florida Program
Program code: 080-11-21-115
Program type: University-based
State: Florida
Address: University of Florida College of Medicine, PO Box 100279,
4037 NW 86 TR, Gainesville, FL 32610-0279
Phone: (352) 594-1925
Fax: (352) 594-1926
Percentage of IMGs in the program: 15%
Minimum USMLE Step 1 Score Requirement: 240
Minimum USMLE Step 2 Score Requirement: 240
Attempts on any step: Must pass on first attempt
CS required at time of application: Yes including ECFMG certificate
USCE Requirement: Yes
Cut-Off time since graduation: 3 years
Program offers couple match: Yes
Visas Sponsored or accepted: J1 visa

Georgia

Emory University Dermatology Residency Program

Specialty: Dermatology
Program name: Emory University Program
Program code: 080-12-21-028
NRMP Code: 1113080A0
Program type: University-based
State: Georgia
Address: Emory University School of Medicine, Department of Dermatology 1st Fl,

> 1525 Clifton Rd, Atlanta, GA 30322

Phone: (404) 727-3669
Fax: (404) 727-5874
Percentage of IMGs in the program: 10%
Minimum USMLE Step 1 Score Requirement: No limits set
Minimum USMLE Step 2 Score Requirement: No limits set
Attempts on any step: No limits set
CS required at time of application: Yes including ECFMG exam
USCE Requirement: Yes
Cut-Off time since graduation: No limits set
Program offers couple match: Yes
Visas Sponsored or accepted: J1 visa and H1b visa

Medical College of Georgia Dermatology Residency Program

Specialty: Dermatology
Program name: Medical College of Georgia Program
Program code: 080-12-11-029
NRMP Code: 1985080A0
Program type: University-based
State: Georgia
Address: Georgia Regents University MCG, Division of Dermatology (FH-100),
1004 Chafee Ave, Augusta, GA 30912
Phone: (706) 721-6231
Fax: (706) 721-6220
Percentage of IMGs in the program: 0%
Minimum USMLE Step 1 Score Requirement: 230
Minimum USMLE Step 2 Score Requirement: 230
Attempts on any step: Must pass on first attempt including CS exam
CS required at time of application: Yes including ECFMG certificate
USCE Requirement: Yes, 3 months
Cut-Off time since graduation: 3 years
Program offers couple match: Yes
Visas Sponsored or accepted: J1 visa

Illinois

Southern Illinois University Dermatology Residency Program

Specialty: Dermatology
Program name: Southern Illinois University Program
Program code: 080-16-21-118
NRMP Code: 2922080C0
Program type: University-based
State: Illinois
Address: Southern Illinois University School of Medicine, PO Box 19644 Suite 2300,
        751 N Rutledge St, Springfield, IL 62794-9644
Phone: (217) 545-5465
Fax: (217) 545-4485
Percentage of IMGs in the program: 0%
Minimum USMLE Step 1 Score Requirement: 220
Minimum USMLE Step 2 Score Requirement: 220
Attempts on any step: No limits set
CS required at time of application: No
USCE Requirement: Yes

Cut-Off time since graduation: 2 years
Program offers couple match: Yes
Visas Sponsored or accepted: J1 visa

Loyola University Dermatology Residency Program

Specialty: Dermatology
Program name: Loyola University Program
Program code: 080-16-12-135
NRMP Code: 1170080A0
Program type: University-based
State: Illinois
Address: Loyola University Medical Center, Building 54 Room 136,
        2160 S First Ave, Maywood, IL 60153
Phone: (708) 216-4807
Fax: (708) 216-2444
Percentage of IMGs in the program: 20%
Minimum USMLE Step 1 Score Requirement: 230
Minimum USMLE Step 2 Score Requirement: 230
Attempts on any step: Must pass on first attempt including CS exam
CS required at time of application: Yes including ECFMG certificate
USCE Requirement: None
Cut-Off time since graduation: 4 years
Program offers couple match: Yes

University of Illinois College of Medicine at Chicago Dermatology Residency Program

Specialty: Dermatology
Program name: University of Illinois College of Medicine at Chicago Program
Program code: 080-16-21-034
Program type: University-based
State: Illinois
Address: University of Illinois Medical Center, M/C 624 Rm 380 910 CME,
          808 S Wood St, Chicago, IL 60612-7307
Phone: (312) 413-7767
Fax: (312) 996-1188
Percentage of IMGs in the program: 0%
Minimum USMLE Step 1 Score Requirement: 210
Minimum USMLE Step 2 Score Requirement: 220
Attempts on any step: Must pass on first attempt including CS exam
CS required at time of application: Yes including ECFMG certificate
USCE Requirement: None
Cut-Off time since graduation: 5 years
Program offers couple match: yes
Visas Sponsored or accepted: J1 visa

McGaw Medical Center of Northwestern University Dermatology Residency Program

Specialty: Dermatology
Program name: McGaw Medical Center of Northwestern University Program
Program code: 080-16-21-031
NRMP Code: 2247080A0
Program type: University-based
State: Illinois
Address: Northwestern University McGaw Medical Center,
    Department of Dermatology Suite 1600,
    676 N St Clair St, Chicago, IL 60611-2997
Phone: (312) 695-7932
Fax: (312) 695-0664
Percentage of IMGs in the program: 0%
Minimum USMLE Step 1 Score Requirement: 205
Minimum USMLE Step 2 Score Requirement: 205
Attempts on any step: No limits set
CS required at time of application: No
USCE Requirement: None

Cut-Off time since graduation: No limits set
Program offers couple match: Yes
Visas Sponsored or accepted: J1 visa and H1b visa

John H Stroger Hospital of Cook County Dermatology Residency Program

Specialty: Dermatology
Program name: John H Stroger Hospital of Cook County Program
Program code: 080-16-12-030
State: Illinois
Address: Stroger Hospital of Cook County, Administration Building Room 519,
          1900 W Polk St, Chicago, IL 60612-9985
Phone: (312) 864-4478
Fax: (312) 864-9663
Percentage of IMGs in the program: 10%
Minimum USMLE Step 1 Score Requirement: 230
Minimum USMLE Step 2 Score Requirement: 230
Attempts on any step: No limits set
CS required at time of application: No
USCE Requirement: Yes
Cut-Off time since graduation: No limits set

Program offers couple match: No
Visas Sponsored or accepted: J1 visa and H1b visa

University of Chicago Dermatology Residency Program

Specialty: Dermatology
Program name: University of Chicago Program
Program code: 080-16-11-033
NRMP Code: 1160080A0
Program type: University-based
State: Illinois
Address: University of Chicago Hospitals, Section of Dermatology MC 5067,
          5841 S Maryland Ave, Chicago, IL 60637-1470
Phone: (773) 702-0549
Fax: (773) 702-8398
Percentage of IMGs in the program: 0%
Minimum USMLE Step 1 Score Requirement: 225
Minimum USMLE Step 2 Score Requirement: 225
Attempts on any step: No limits set
CS required at time of application: No
USCE Requirement: Yes
Cut-Off time since graduation: No limits set
Program offers couple match: Yes
Visas Sponsored or accepted: J1 visa

Rush University Medical Center Dermatology Residency Program

Specialty: Dermatology
Program name: Rush University Medical Center Program
Program code: 080-16-11-032
NRMP Code: 1147080A0
Program type: University-based
State: Illinois
Address: Rush University Medical Center, 220 Annex Building,
        1653 W Congress Pkwy, Chicago, IL 60612
Phone: (312) 942-6097
Fax: (312) 942-7778
Percentage of IMGs in the program: 0%
Minimum USMLE Step 1 Score Requirement: No limits set
Minimum USMLE Step 2 Score Requirement: No limits set
Attempts on any step: Maximum of 2 attempts on each step
CS required at time of application: Yes including ECFMG certificate
USCE Requirement: Yes
Cut-Off time since graduation: 5 years
Program offers couple match: Yes
Visas Sponsored or accepted: No visa

Indiana

Indiana University School of Medicine Dermatology Residency Program

Specialty: Dermatology
Program name: Indiana University School of Medicine Program
Program code: 080-17-21-035
NRMP Code: 1187080C0
Program type: Community-based university affiliated hospital
State: Indiana
Address: Indiana University Medical Center, EH 139,
        545 Barnhill Dr, Indianapolis, IN 46202-5267
Phone: (317) 278-6833
Fax: (317) 274-3700
Percentage of IMGs in the program: 10%
Minimum USMLE Step 1 Score Requirement: 220

Minimum USMLE Step 2 Score Requirement:
220
Attempts on any step: No limits set
CS required at time of application: Yes
including ECFMG certificate
USCE Requirement: None
Cut-Off time since graduation: No limits set
Program offers couple match: Yes
Visas Sponsored or accepted: No visa

Iowa

University of Iowa Hospitals and Clinics Dermatology Residency Program

Specialty: Dermatology
Program name: University of Iowa Hospitals and Clinics Program
Program code: 080-18-21-036
State: Iowa
Address: University of Iowa Hospitals and Clinics, Department of Dermatology,
        200 Hawkins Dr, Iowa City, IA 52242-1090
Phone: (319) 356-1694
Fax: (319) 356-0349

Percentage of IMGs in the program: 0%
Minimum USMLE Step 1 Score Requirement: 225
Minimum USMLE Step 2 Score Requirement: 225
Attempts on any step: Must pass on first attempt
CS required at time of application:
USCE Requirement: Yes
Cut-Off time since graduation: 5 years
Program offers couple match: No
Visas Sponsored or accepted: J1 visa

Kansas

University of Kansas School of Medicine Dermatology Residency Program

Specialty: Dermatology
Program name: University of Kansas School of Medicine Program
Program code: 080-19-11-037
Program type: University-based
State: Kansas
Address: University of Kansas Medical Center, MS2025 Rm 4010 Wescoe,

3901 Rainbow Blvd, Kansas City, KS 66160-7319
Phone: (913) 588-3840
Fax: (913) 588-8300
Percentage of IMGs in the program: 8%
Minimum USMLE Step 1 Score Requirement: 230
Minimum USMLE Step 2 Score Requirement: 230
Attempts on any step: No limits set
CS required at time of application:
USCE Requirement: Yes including ECFMG certificate
Cut-Off time since graduation: No limits set
Program offers couple match: Yes
Visas Sponsored or accepted: J1 visa and H1b visa

Kentucky

University of Louisville Dermatology Residency Program

Specialty: Dermatology
Program name: University of Louisville Program
Program code: 080-20-21-038

NRMP Code:
Program type: University-based
State: Kentucky
Address: University of Louisville Health Science
Center, Division of Dermatology Fl 2A,
            310 E Broadway, Louisville, KY 40292
Phone: (502) 852-7287
Fax: (502) 852-4720
Percentage of IMGs in the program: 0%
Minimum USMLE Step 1 Score Requirement:
No limits set
Minimum USMLE Step 2 Score Requirement:
No limits set
Attempts on any step: No limits set
CS required at time of application: Yes
USCE Requirement: None
Cut-Off time since graduation: No limits set
Program offers couple match: Yes
Visas Sponsored or accepted: No visa

Louisiana

Louisiana State University Dermatology Residency Program

Specialty: Dermatology

Program name: Louisiana State University Program
Program code: 080-21-21-109
Program type: University-based
State: Louisiana
Address: LSU Health Science Center New Orleans, Department of Dermatology Suite 639, 1542 Tulane Ave, New Orleans, LA 70112-2822
Phone: (504) 568-7110
Fax: (504) 568-2170
Percentage of IMGs in the program: 0%
Minimum USMLE Step 1 Score Requirement: No limits set
Minimum USMLE Step 2 Score Requirement: No limits set
Attempts on any step: No limits set
CS required at time of application: Yes including ECFMG certificate
USCE Requirement: Yes
Cut-Off time since graduation: No limits set
Program offers couple match: Yes
Visas Sponsored or accepted: J1 visa

Tulane University Dermatology Residency Program

Specialty: Dermatology
Program name: Tulane University Program
Program code: 080-21-21-108

NRMP Code:
Program type:
State: Louisiana
Address: Tulane University Health Sciences Center, #8036,
          1430 Tulane Ave, New Orleans, LA 70112
Phone: (504) 988-5126
Fax: (504) 988-7382
Percentage of IMGs in the program: 0%
Minimum USMLE Step 1 Score Requirement: No limits set
Minimum USMLE Step 2 Score Requirement: No limits set
Attempts on any step: No limits set
CS required at time of application: No
USCE Requirement: None
Cut-Off time since graduation: No limits set
Program offers couple match: Yes
Visas Sponsored or accepted: No visa

Maryland

University of Maryland Dermatology Residency Program

Specialty: Dermatology
Program name: University of Maryland Program

Program code: 080-23-21-041
Program type: University-based
State: Maryland
Address: University of Maryland Medical System, Department of Dermatology Suite 240, 419 W Redwood St, Baltimore, MD 21201
Phone: (410) 328-5766
Fax: (410) 328-0098
Percentage of IMGs in the program: 0%
Minimum USMLE Step 1 Score Requirement: 235
Minimum USMLE Step 2 Score Requirement: 235
Attempts on any step: No limits set
CS required at time of application: No
USCE Requirement: Yes
Cut-Off time since graduation: 3 years
Program offers couple match: Yes
Visas Sponsored or accepted: J1 visa

Johns Hopkins University Dermatology Residency Program

Specialty: Dermatology
Program name: Johns Hopkins University Program
Program code: 080-23-21-040
Program type: University-based
State: Maryland

Address: Johns Hopkins Medical Institutions, Suite 211,

        1550 Orleans St, Baltimore, MD 21231

Phone: (410) 955-2400

Fax: (410) 955-8645

Percentage of IMGs in the program: 0%

Minimum USMLE Step 1 Score Requirement: No limits set

Minimum USMLE Step 2 Score Requirement: No limits set

Attempts on any step: No limits set

CS required at time of application: Yes including ECFMG certificate

USCE Requirement: None

Cut-Off time since graduation: No limits set

Program offers couple match: Yes

Visas Sponsored or accepted: J1 visa

Massachusetts

University of Massachusetts Dermatology Residency Program

Specialty: Dermatology

Program name: University of Massachusetts Program
Program code: 080-24-21-114
Program type: University-based
State: Massachusetts
Address: UMass Memorial Health Care, Division of Dermatology,
        281 Lincoln St, Worcester, MA 01605
Phone: (508) 334-5971
Fax: (508) 334-5981
Percentage of IMGs in the program: 0%
Minimum USMLE Step 1 Score Requirement: 210
Minimum USMLE Step 2 Score Requirement: 210
Attempts on any step: No limits set
CS required at time of application: No
USCE Requirement: None
Cut-Off time since graduation: No limits set
Program offers couple match: Yes
Visas Sponsored or accepted: J1 visa and H1b visa

Massachusetts General Hospital/Beth Israel Deaconess Medical Center/Brigham and Women's Hospital Dermatology Residency Program

Specialty: Dermatology
Program name: Massachusetts General Hospital/Beth Israel Deaconess Medical Center/Brigham and Women's Hospital Program
Program code: 080-24-31-043
State: Massachusetts
Address: Massachusetts General Hospital, Bartlett Hall 616,
        55 Fruit St, Boston, MA 02114
Phone: (617) 726-5254
Fax: (617) 726-1875
Percentage of IMGs in the program: 6%
Minimum USMLE Step 1 Score Requirement: 215
Minimum USMLE Step 2 Score Requirement: 215
Attempts on any step: No limits set
CS required at time of application: No
USCE Requirement: Yes
Cut-Off time since graduation: No limits set
Program offers couple match: No
Visas Sponsored or accepted: J1 visa and H1b visa

Tufts Medical Center Dermatology Residency Program

Specialty: Dermatology
Program name: Tufts Medical Center Program

Program code: 080-24-21-141
State: Massachusetts
Address: Tufts Medical Center, Department of Dermatology #114,
            800 Washington St, Boston, MA 02111
Phone: (617) 636-7480
Fax: (617) 636-9169
Percentage of IMGs in the program: 20%
Minimum USMLE Step 1 Score Requirement: 230
Minimum USMLE Step 2 Score Requirement: 230
Attempts on any step: Must pass on first attempt
CS required at time of application: Yes including ECFMG certificate
USCE Requirement: None
Cut-Off time since graduation: 10 years
Program offers couple match: No
Visas Sponsored or accepted: J1 visa

Boston Medical Center Dermatology Residency Program

Specialty: Dermatology
Program name: Boston Medical Center Program
Program code: 080-24-21-044
State: Massachusetts

Address: Boston University Medical Center, Department of Dermatology J-202,
609 Albany St, Boston, MA 02118-2394
Phone: (617) 414-1366
Fax: (617) 414-1363
Percentage of IMGs in the program: 6%
Minimum USMLE Step 1 Score Requirement: No limits set
Minimum USMLE Step 2 Score Requirement: No limits set
Attempts on any step: No limits set
CS required at time of application: Yes including ECFMG Certificate
USCE Requirement: None
Cut-Off time since graduation: No limits set
Program offers couple match: No
Visas Sponsored or accepted: J1 visa

Michigan

Wayne State University School of Medicine Dermatology Residency Program

Specialty: Dermatology
Program name: Wayne State University School of Medicine Program
Program code: 080-25-13-139
Program type: University-based
State: Michigan
Address: Wayne State University, Dermatology Suite 300,

18100 Oakwood Blvd, Detroit, MI 48124
Phone: (313) 429-7843
Fax: (313) 429-7931
Percentage of IMGs in the program: 0%
Minimum USMLE Step 1 Score Requirement: No limits set
Minimum USMLE Step 2 Score Requirement: No limits set
Attempts on any step: No limits set
CS required at time of application: Yes including ECFMG certificate
USCE Requirement: None
Cut-Off time since graduation: No limits set
Program offers couple match: Yes
Visas Sponsored or accepted: No visa

Henry Ford Hospital/Wayne State University Dermatology Residency Program

Specialty: Dermatology
Program name: Henry Ford Hospital/Wayne State University Program
Program code: 080-25-12-046
Program type: Community-based university affiliated hospital
State: Michigan
Address: Henry Ford Hospital/Wayne State University, Department of Dermatology Suite 800,

      3031 W Grand Blvd, Detroit, MI 48202
Phone: (313) 916-2171
Fax: (313) 916-2093
Percentage of IMGs in the program: 0%
Minimum USMLE Step 1 Score Requirement: No limits set
Minimum USMLE Step 2 Score Requirement: No limits set
Attempts on any step: No limits set
CS required at time of application: No
USCE Requirement: Yes
Cut-Off time since graduation: No limits set
Program offers couple match: Yes
Visas Sponsored or accepted: J1 visa

University of Michigan Dermatology Residency Program

Specialty: Dermatology
Program name: University of Michigan Program
Program code: 080-25-31-045
Program type: University-based
State: Michigan
Address: University of Michigan Hospitals, 1910 Taubman Center 5314,
　　　　1500 E Medical Center Dr, Ann Arbor, MI 48109
Phone: (734) 936-6674
Fax: (734) 936-6395
Percentage of IMGs in the program: 0%
Minimum USMLE Step 1 Score Requirement: 220
Minimum USMLE Step 2 Score Requirement: 220
Attempts on any step: No limits set
CS required at time of application: Yes
USCE Requirement: None
Cut-Off time since graduation: No limits set
Program offers couple match: Yes
Visas Sponsored or accepted: J1 visa

Minnesota

Mayo Clinic College of Medicine (Rochester) Dermatology Residency Program

Specialty: Dermatology
Program name: Mayo Clinic College of Medicine (Rochester) Program
Program code: 080-26-21-049
NRMP Code: 1328080C0
Program type: University-based
State: Minnesota
Address: Mayo Clinic, Department of Dermatology,
    200 First St SW, Rochester, MN 55905
Phone: (507) 284-5997
Fax: (507) 284-2072
Percentage of IMGs in the program: 0%
Minimum USMLE Step 1 Score Requirement: No limits set
Minimum USMLE Step 2 Score Requirement: No limits set
Attempts on any step: Maximum of 3 attempts on each step including CS exam
CS required at time of application: No
USCE Requirement: None
Cut-Off time since graduation: No limits set
Program offers couple match: Yes

Visas Sponsored or accepted: J1 visa and H1b visa

University of Minnesota Dermatology Residency Program

Specialty: Dermatology
Program name: University of Minnesota Program
Program code: 080-26-31-048
Program type: University-based
State: Minnesota
Address: University of Minnesota Medical Center, Department of Dermatology MMC 98,
        420 Delaware St SE, Minneapolis, MN 55455-0392
Phone: (612) 624-9964
Fax: (612) 624-6678
Percentage of IMGs in the program: 5%
Minimum USMLE Step 1 Score Requirement: 230
Minimum USMLE Step 2 Score Requirement: 230
Attempts on any step: No limits set
CS required at time of application: No
USCE Requirement: None
Cut-Off time since graduation: No limits set
Program offers couple match: Yes
Visas Sponsored or accepted: J1 visa

Mississippi

University of Mississippi School of Medicine Dermatology Residency Program

Specialty: Dermatology
Program name: University of Mississippi School of Medicine Program
Program code: 080-27-00-001
Program type: University-based
State: Mississippi
Address: University of Mississippi Medical Center, Dermatology Program,
          2500 N State St, Jackson, MS 39216
Phone: (601) 334-6007
Fax: (601) 984-5085
Percentage of IMGs in the program: 0%
Minimum USMLE Step 1 Score Requirement: 230
Minimum USMLE Step 2 Score Requirement: 230
Attempts on any step: Must pass on first attempt including CS exam
CS required at time of application: Yes including ECFMG certificate
USCE Requirement: Yes

Cut-Off time since graduation: 5 years
Program offers couple match: No
Visas Sponsored or accepted: No visa

Missouri

St Louis University School of Medicine Dermatology Residency Program

Specialty: Dermatology
Program name: St Louis University School of Medicine Program
Program code: 080-28-21-116
Program type: University-based
State: Missouri
Address: St Louis University School of Medicine, Department of Dermatology,
          1402 S Grand Blvd, St Louis, MO 63104
Phone: (314) 256-3435
Fax: (314) 256-3431
Percentage of IMGs in the program: 0%
Minimum USMLE Step 1 Score Requirement: 220

Minimum USMLE Step 2 Score Requirement: 220
Attempts on any step: No limits set
CS required at time of application: No
USCE Requirement: Yes
Cut-Off time since graduation: No limits set
Program offers couple match: No
Visas Sponsored or accepted: J1 visa

Washington University/B-JH/SLCH Consortium Dermatology Residency Program

Specialty: Dermatology
Program name: Washington University/B-JH/SLCH Consortium Program
Program code: 080-28-21-051
State: Missouri
Address: Washington University Medical Center, Division of Dermatology Campus Box 8123,
        660 S Euclid Ave, St Louis, MO 63110
Phone: (314) 454-8622
Fax: (314) 454-5928
Percentage of IMGs in the program: 0%
Minimum USMLE Step 1 Score Requirement: 240
Minimum USMLE Step 2 Score Requirement: 240

Attempts on any step: Must pass on first attempt on any step including CS exam
CS required at time of application: Yes including ECFMG certificate
USCE Requirement: Yes
Cut-Off time since graduation: No limits set
Program offers couple match: Yes
Visas Sponsored or accepted: No visa

University of Missouri-Columbia Dermatology Residency Program

Specialty: Dermatology
Program name: University of Missouri-Columbia Program
Program code: 080-28-21-050
Program type: University-based
State: Missouri
Address: University of Missouri Hospitals and Clinics, Dermatology Room MA111 HSC,
              One Hospital Dr, Columbia, MO 65212
Phone: (573) 882-9485
Fax: (573) 884-5947
Percentage of IMGs in the program: 0%
Minimum USMLE Step 1 Score Requirement: No limits set
Minimum USMLE Step 2 Score Requirement: No limits set
Attempts on any step: No limits set

CS required at time of application: Yes including ECFMG certificate
USCE Requirement: None
Cut-Off time since graduation: No limits set
Program offers couple match: Yes
Visas Sponsored or accepted: J1 visa and H1b visa

New Hampshire

Dartmouth-Hitchcock Medical Center Dermatology Residency Program

Specialty: Dermatology
Program name: Dartmouth-Hitchcock Medical Center Program
Program code: 080-32-21-053
Program type: University-based
State: New Hampshire
Address: Dartmouth-Hitchcock Medical Center, Section of Dermatology,
        One Medical Center Dr, Lebanon, NH 03756
Phone: (603) 650-3156
Fax: (603) 650-3172

Percentage of IMGs in the program: 18%
Minimum USMLE Step 1 Score Requirement: 220
Minimum USMLE Step 2 Score Requirement: 220
Attempts on any step: No limits set
CS required at time of application: Yes
USCE Requirement: Yes
Cut-Off time since graduation: No limits set
Program offers couple match: Yes
Visas Sponsored or accepted: J1 visa

New Jersey

Rutgers Robert Wood Johnson Medical School Dermatology Residency Program

Specialty: Dermatology
Program name: Rutgers Robert Wood Johnson Medical School Program
Program code: 080-33-31-128
State: New Jersey
Address: UMDNJ-Robert Wood Johnson Medical School,

Department of Dermatology Suite 2400,

1 World's Fair Dr, Somerset, NJ 08873
Phone: (732) 235-7765
Fax: (732) 235-6568
Percentage of IMGs in the program: 15%
Minimum USMLE Step 1 Score Requirement: No limits set
Minimum USMLE Step 2 Score Requirement: No limits set
Attempts on any step: No limits set
CS required at time of application: Yes including ECFMG certificate
USCE Requirement: None
Cut-Off time since graduation: No limits set
Program offers couple match: No
Visas Sponsored or accepted: No visa

Rutgers New Jersey Medical School Dermatology Residency Program

Specialty: Dermatology
Program name: Rutgers New Jersey Medical School Program
Program code: 080-33-21-107
State: New Jersey
Address: Rutgers New Jersey Medical School, Department of Dermatology,

185 S Orange Ave, Newark, NJ 07103
Phone: (973) 972-6884

Fax: (973) 972-5877
Percentage of IMGs in the program: 0%
Minimum USMLE Step 1 Score Requirement:
No limits set
Minimum USMLE Step 2 Score Requirement:
No limits set
Attempts on any step: No limits set
CS required at time of application: No
USCE Requirement: None
Cut-Off time since graduation: No limits set
Program offers couple match: Yes
Visas Sponsored or accepted: No visa

Cooper Medical School of Rowan University/Cooper University Hospital Dermatology Residency Program

Specialty: Dermatology
Program name: Cooper Medical School of
Rowan University/Cooper University Hospital
Program
Program code: 080-33-21-117
NRMP Code: 1380080A0
Program type: University-based
State: New Jersey
Address: Cooper Hospital-University Medical
Center, Division of Dermatology Suite 504,
      3 Cooper Plaza, Camden, NJ 08103
Phone: (856) 342-2030

Fax: (856) 966-0735
Percentage of IMGs in the program: 0%
Minimum USMLE Step 1 Score Requirement:
No limits set
Minimum USMLE Step 2 Score Requirement:
No limits set
Attempts on any step: No limits set
CS required at time of application: Yes
including ECFMG certificate
USCE Requirement: None
Cut-Off time since graduation: 3 years
Program offers couple match: No
Visas Sponsored or accepted: J1 visa

New Mexico

University of New Mexico Dermatology Residency Program

Specialty: Dermatology
Program name: University of New Mexico
Program
Program code: 080-34-21-054
State: New Mexico
Address: University of New Mexico Health
Science Center,

Department of Dermatology MSC 07 4240,

1021 Medical Arts Ave NE, Albuquerque, NM 87131-5231

Phone: (505) 272-6000
Fax: (505) 272-6003
Percentage of IMGs in the program: 0%
Minimum USMLE Step 1 Score Requirement: 235
Minimum USMLE Step 2 Score Requirement: 235
Attempts on any step: No limits set
CS required at time of application: Yes
USCE Requirement: None
Cut-Off time since graduation: No limits set
Program offers couple match: Yes
Visas Sponsored or accepted: J1 visa

New York

SUNY at Stony Brook Dermatology Residency Program

Specialty: Dermatology
Program name: SUNY at Stony Brook Program

Program code: 080-35-21-113
State: New York
Address: SUNY Stony Brook University,
Department of Dermatology,
        Health Science Center T-16 Rm 060,
Stony Brook, NY 11794-8165
Phone: (631) 444-3843
Fax: (631) 444-3844
Percentage of IMGs in the program: 0%
Minimum USMLE Step 1 Score Requirement:
220
Minimum USMLE Step 2 Score Requirement:
220
Attempts on any step: Must pass on first
attempt
CS required at time of application: Yes
including ECFMG certificate
USCE Requirement: None
Cut-Off time since graduation: No limits set
Program offers couple match: No
Visas Sponsored or accepted: J1 visa

University of Rochester
Dermatology Residency Program

Specialty: Dermatology
Program name: University of Rochester
Program
Program code: 080-35-21-102
Program type: University-based
State: New York

Address: University of Rochester Medical Center, Box 697,
            601 Elmwood Ave, Rochester, NY 14642
Phone: (585) 275-0193
Fax: (585) 275-0022
Percentage of IMGs in the program: 0%
Minimum USMLE Step 1 Score Requirement: 240
Minimum USMLE Step 2 Score Requirement: 240
Attempts on any step: No limits set
CS required at time of application: Yes including ECFMG certificate
USCE Requirement: 1 month
Cut-Off time since graduation: No limits set
Program offers couple match: Yes
Visas Sponsored or accepted: J1 visa

St Luke's-Roosevelt Hospital Center Dermatology Residency Program

Specialty: Dermatology
Program name: St Luke's-Roosevelt Hospital Center Program
Program code: 080-35-21-124
NRMP Code: 2070080A0
Program type: Community-based university affiliated hospital
State: New York

Address: St Luke's-Roosevelt Hospital Center, Department of Dermatology Suite 11B,
1090 Amsterdam Ave, New York, NY 10025
Phone: (212) 523-3812
Fax: (212) 523-3808
Percentage of IMGs in the program: 20%
Minimum USMLE Step 1 Score Requirement: No limits set
Minimum USMLE Step 2 Score Requirement: No limits set
Attempts on any step: No limits set
CS required at time of application: Yes including ECFMG certificate
USCE Requirement: None
Cut-Off time since graduation: No limits set
Program offers couple match: Yes
Visas Sponsored or accepted: J1 visa

New York Presbyterian Hospital (Columbia Campus) Dermatology Residency Program

Specialty: Dermatology
Program name: New York Presbyterian Hospital (Columbia Campus) Program
Program code: 080-35-21-104
State: New York

Address: New York Presbyterian Hospital-
Columbia, Department of Dermatology 12th
Floor,

161 Fort Washington Ave, New York,
NY 10032
Phone: (212) 305-5317
Fax: (212) 342-4571
Percentage of IMGs in the program: 0%
Minimum USMLE Step 1 Score Requirement:
No limits set
Minimum USMLE Step 2 Score Requirement:
No limits set
Attempts on any step: No limits set
CS required at time of application: No
USCE Requirement: None
Cut-Off time since graduation: No limits set
Program offers couple match: No
Visas Sponsored or accepted: No visa

New York University School of Medicine Dermatology Residency Program

Specialty: Dermatology
Program name: New York University School of
Medicine Program
Program code: 080-35-21-064
Program type: University-based
State: New York
Address: New York University Medical Center,

Ambulatory Care Ctr Dermatology Pgm 11th Floor,
240 E 38th St, New York, NY 10016
Phone: (212) 263-3722
Fax: (212) 263-8752
Percentage of IMGs in the program: 5%
Minimum USMLE Step 1 Score Requirement: No limits set
Minimum USMLE Step 2 Score Requirement: No limits set
Attempts on any step: No limits set
CS required at time of application: Yes including ECFMG certificate
USCE Requirement: None
Cut-Off time since graduation: No limits set
Program offers couple match: Yes
Visas Sponsored or accepted: J1 visa and H1b visa

New York Medical College (Metropolitan) Dermatology Residency Program

Specialty: Dermatology
Program name: New York Medical College (Metropolitan) Program
Program code: 080-35-21-063
Program type: University-based
State: New York

Address: Metropolitan Hospital Center, Department of Dermatology Room 1208, 1901 First Ave, New York, NY 10029
Phone: (212) 423-7467
Fax: (212) 423-8464
Percentage of IMGs in the program: 25%
Minimum USMLE Step 1 Score Requirement: 225
Minimum USMLE Step 2 Score Requirement: 225
Attempts on any step: Must pass on first attempt including CS exam
CS required at time of application: Yes including ECFMG certificate
USCE Requirement: None
Cut-Off time since graduation: 3 years
Program offers couple match: No
Visas Sponsored or accepted: J1 visa and H1b visa

New York Presbyterian Hospital (Cornell Campus) Dermatology Residency Program

Specialty: Dermatology
Program name: New York Presbyterian Hospital (Cornell Campus) Program
Program code: 080-35-21-062
State: New York

Address: New York Presbyterian Hospital-Cornell, Dermatology Pgm 9th Floor,
1305 York Ave, New York, NY 10021
Phone: (646) 962-7275
Fax: (646) 962-0040
Percentage of IMGs in the program: 0%
Minimum USMLE Step 1 Score Requirement: 210
Minimum USMLE Step 2 Score Requirement: 210
Attempts on any step: No limits set
CS required at time of application: No
USCE Requirement: None
Cut-Off time since graduation: No limits set
Program offers couple match: Yes
Visas Sponsored or accepted: J1 visa

Icahn School of Medicine at Mount Sinai Dermatology Residency Program

Specialty: Dermatology
Program name: Icahn School of Medicine at Mount Sinai Program
Program code: 080-35-21-061
NRMP Code: 1490080A0
Program type: University-based
State: New York
Address: Mount Sinai Medical Center, Department of Dermatology Box 1047,

One Gustave L Levy Pl, New York, NY
10029-6594
Phone: (212) 659-9530
Fax: (212) 348-7434
Percentage of IMGs in the program: 0%
Minimum USMLE Step 1 Score Requirement:
230
Minimum USMLE Step 2 Score Requirement:
230
Attempts on any step: Must pass on first
attempt on any step
CS required at time of application: Yes
including ECFMG Certificate
USCE Requirement: Yes
Cut-Off time since graduation: No limits set
Program offers couple match: No
Visas Sponsored or accepted: No visa

SUNY Health Science Center at Brooklyn Dermatology Residency Program

Specialty: Dermatology
Program name: SUNY Health Science Center at
Brooklyn Program
Program code: 080-35-21-065
NRMP Code: 1426080A0
Program type: University-based
State: New York

Address: SUNY Downstate Medical Center, Department of Dermatology,
        450 Clarkson Ave, Brooklyn, NY 11203
Phone: (718) 270-1229
Fax: (718) 270-2794
Percentage of IMGs in the program: 8%
Minimum USMLE Step 1 Score Requirement: 230
Minimum USMLE Step 2 Score Requirement: 230
Attempts on any step: No limits set
CS required at time of application: Yes including ECFMG certificate
USCE Requirement: None
Cut-Off time since graduation: No limits set
Program offers couple match: No
Visas Sponsored or accepted: No visa

Albert Einstein College of Medicine Dermatology Residency Program

Specialty: Dermatology
Program name: Albert Einstein College of Medicine Program
Program code: 080-35-31-058
NRMP Code: 3153080A0
Program type: University-based
State: New York
Address: Montefiore Medical Center, Division of Dermatology,

111 E 210th St, Bronx, NY 10467-2490
Phone: (718) 920-2680
Fax: (718) 944-4219
Percentage of IMGs in the program: 8%
Minimum USMLE Step 1 Score Requirement: 215
Minimum USMLE Step 2 Score Requirement: 215
Attempts on any step: No limits set
CS required at time of application: No
USCE Requirement: Yes
Cut-Off time since graduation: No limits set
Program offers couple match: Yes
Visas Sponsored or accepted: No visa

North Carolina

Wake Forest University School of Medicine Dermatology Residency Program

Specialty: Dermatology
Program name: Wake Forest University School of Medicine Program
Program code: 080-36-21-110
Program type: University-based

State: North Carolina
Address: Wake Forest Baptist Medical center, Department of Dermatology,
          Medical Center Blvd, Winston-Salem, NC 27157
Phone: (336) 716-2768
Fax: (336) 716-7732
Percentage of IMGs in the program: 0%
Minimum USMLE Step 1 Score Requirement: No limits set
Minimum USMLE Step 2 Score Requirement: No limits set
Attempts on any step: Maximum of 3 attempts on each step including CS exam
CS required at time of application: No
USCE Requirement: No
Cut-Off time since graduation: No limits set
Program offers couple match: No
Visas Sponsored or accepted: J1 visa

Vidant Medical Center/East Carolina University Dermatology Residency Program

Specialty: Dermatology
Program name: Vidant Medical Center/East Carolina University Program
Program code: 080-36-13-132
Program type: University-based
State: North Carolina

Address: Brody School of Medicine ECU, Brody 3E-117,

       600 Moye Blvd, Greenville, NC 27834

Phone: (252) 744-2555
Fax: (252) 744-3047
Percentage of IMGs in the program: 0%
Minimum USMLE Step 1 Score Requirement: No limits set
Minimum USMLE Step 2 Score Requirement: No limits set
Attempts on any step: No limits set
CS required at time of application: No
USCE Requirement: None
Cut-Off time since graduation: No limits set
Program offers couple match: Yes
Visas Sponsored or accepted: J1 visa

Duke University Hospital Dermatology Residency Program

Specialty: Dermatology
Program name: Duke University Hospital Program
Program code: 080-36-21-067
Program type: University-based
State: North Carolina
Address: Duke University Medical Center, Box 3822 DUMC,

       40 Duke Medical Circle, Durham, NC 27710

Phone: (919) 694-6973
Fax: (919) 684-9577
Percentage of IMGs in the program: 0%
Minimum USMLE Step 1 Score Requirement:
No limits set
Minimum USMLE Step 2 Score Requirement:
No limits set
Attempts on any step: No limits set
CS required at time of application: No
USCE Requirement: None
Cut-Off time since graduation: No limits set
Program offers couple match: No
Visas Sponsored or accepted: J1 visa and H1b
visa

University of North Carolina Hospitals Dermatology Residency Program

Specialty: Dermatology
Program name: University of North Carolina
Hospitals Program
Program code: 080-36-11-066
Program type: University-based
State: North Carolina
Address: University of North Carolina Hospitals,
        Department of Dermatology CB#7715t
Suite 400,
        410 Market St, Chapel Hill, NC 27516
Phone: (919) 843-5539

Fax: (919) 966-6460
Percentage of IMGs in the program: 5%
Minimum USMLE Step 1 Score Requirement:
No limits set
Minimum USMLE Step 2 Score Requirement:
No limits set
Attempts on any step: No limits set
CS required at time of application: No
USCE Requirement: None
Cut-Off time since graduation: No limits set
Program offers couple match: Yes
Visas Sponsored or accepted: J1 visa

Ohio

Wright State University Dermatology Residency Program

Specialty: Dermatology
Program name: Wright State University
Program
Program code: 080-38-21-073
Program type: University-based
State: Ohio
Address: Wright State University, Department
of Dermatology,
          PO Box 927, Dayton, OH 45401-0927

Phone: (937) 245-7254
Fax: (937) 245-7927
Percentage of IMGs in the program: 0%
Minimum USMLE Step 1 Score Requirement:
No limits set
Minimum USMLE Step 2 Score Requirement:
No limits set
Attempts on any step: No limits set
CS required at time of application: Yes
including ECFMG certificate
USCE Requirement: None
Cut-Off time since graduation: No limits set
Program offers couple match: No
Visas Sponsored or accepted: No visa

Ohio State University Hospital Dermatology Residency Program

Specialty: Dermatology
Program name: Ohio State University Hospital
Program
Program code: 080-38-11-072
NRMP Code: 1566080C0
Program type: University-based
State: Ohio
Address: Ohio State University Medical Center,
Dermatology Division,
          2012 Kenny Rd, Columbus, OH 43221
Phone:(614) 293-4434
Fax: (614) 293-8090

Percentage of IMGs in the program: 0%
Minimum USMLE Step 1 Score Requirement:
No limits set
Minimum USMLE Step 2 Score Requirement:
No limits set
Attempts on any step: Must pass on first
attempt
CS required at time of application: No
USCE Requirement: None
Cut-Off time since graduation: No limits set
Program offers couple match: Yes
Visas Sponsored or accepted: J1 visa

MetroHealth Medical Center/Case Western Reserve University Dermatology Residency Program

Specialty: Dermatology
Program name: MetroHealth Medical
Center/Case Western Reserve University
Program
Program code: 080-38-31-143
Program type: Community-based
State: Ohio
Address: MetroHealth Medical Center,
Dermatology Program,
2500 MetroHealth Dr, Cleveland, OH
44109
Phone: (216) 778-4973
Fax: (216) 778-2397

Percentage of IMGs in the program: 0%
Minimum USMLE Step 1 Score Requirement: 215
Minimum USMLE Step 2 Score Requirement: 215
Attempts on any step: Must pass on first attempt including CS exam
CS required at time of application: Yes
USCE Requirement: 1 month
Cut-Off time since graduation: No limits set
Program offers couple match: Yes
Visas Sponsored or accepted: No visa

Case Western Reserve University/University Hospitals Case Medical Center Dermatology Residency Program

Specialty: Dermatology
Program name: Case Western Reserve University/University Hospitals Case Medical Center Program
Program code: 080-38-21-120
State: Ohio
Address: University Hospitals Case Medical Center, Department of Dermatology,
       11100 Euclid Ave, Cleveland, OH 44106-5028
Phone: (216) 844-5794
Fax: (216) 844-8993

Percentage of IMGs in the program: 0%
Minimum USMLE Step 1 Score Requirement: No limits set
Minimum USMLE Step 2 Score Requirement: No limits set
Attempts on any step: Must pass on first attempt on any step
CS required at time of application: No
USCE Requirement: None
Cut-Off time since graduation: No limits set
Program offers couple match: Yes
Visas Sponsored or accepted: J1 visa

Cleveland Clinic Foundation Dermatology Residency Program

Specialty: Dermatology
Program name: Cleveland Clinic Foundation Program
Program code: 080-38-12-070
NRMP Code: 1968080C0
Program type: University-based
State: Ohio
Address: Cleveland Clinic, Desk A60,
           9500 Euclid Ave, Cleveland, OH 44195-5242
Phone: (216) 444-5933
Fax: (216) 636-5830
Percentage of IMGs in the program: 5%

Minimum USMLE Step 1 Score Requirement:
No limits set
Minimum USMLE Step 2 Score Requirement:
No limits set
Attempts on any step: No limits set
CS required at time of application: No
USCE Requirement: None
Cut-Off time since graduation: No limits set
Program offers couple match: Yes
Visas Sponsored or accepted: J1 visa and H1b
visa

University of Cincinnati Medical Center/College of Medicine Dermatology Residency Program

Specialty: Dermatology
Program name: University of Cincinnati Medical Center/College of Medicine Program
Program code: 080-38-21-068
NRMP Code: 1548080A0
Program type: University-based
State: Ohio
Address: University Hospital University of Cincinnati,
        Department of Dermatology PO Box 670592,
        231 Albert Sabin Way, Cincinnati, OH 45267-0592
Phone: (513) 558-6302

Fax: (513) 558-0198
Percentage of IMGs in the program: 0%
Minimum USMLE Step 1 Score Requirement: No limits set
Minimum USMLE Step 2 Score Requirement: No limits set
Attempts on any step: Must pass on first attempt on any step
CS required at time of application: Yes including ECFMG certificate
USCE Requirement: None
Cut-Off time since graduation: No limits set
Program offers couple match: Yes
Visas Sponsored or accepted: J1 visa

Oklahoma

University of Oklahoma Health Sciences Center Dermatology Residency Program

Specialty: Dermatology
Program name: University of Oklahoma Health Sciences Center Program
Program code: 080-39-21-074

NRMP Code: 1588080A0
Program type: University-based
State: Oklahoma
Address: University of Oklahoma Health Sciences Center, Department of Dermatology, 619 NE 13th St, Oklahoma City, OK 73104
Phone: (405) 271-6110   Ext: 48002
Fax: (405) 271-7216
Percentage of IMGs in the program: 0%
Minimum USMLE Step 1 Score Requirement: 240
Minimum USMLE Step 2 Score Requirement: 240
Attempts on any step: Must pass on first attempt including CS exam
CS required at time of application: No
USCE Requirement: None
Cut-Off time since graduation: No limits set
Program offers couple match: No
Visas Sponsored or accepted: No visa

Oregon

Oregon Health & Science University Dermatology Residency Program

Specialty: Dermatology
Program name: Oregon Health & Science University Program
Program code: 080-40-21-075
Program type: University-based
State: Oregon
Address: Oregon Health & Science University, Center for Health and Healing CH16D, 3303 SW Bond Ave, Portland, OR 97239
Phone: (503) 494-1375
Fax: (503) 494-6844
Percentage of IMGs in the program: 0%
Minimum USMLE Step 1 Score Requirement: No limits set
Minimum USMLE Step 2 Score Requirement: No limits set
Attempts on any step: No limits set
CS required at time of application: No
USCE Requirement: None
Cut-Off time since graduation: No limits set
Program offers couple match: Yes
Visas Sponsored or accepted: No visa

Pennsylvania

UPMC Medical Education Dermatology Residency Program

Specialty: Dermatology
Program name: UPMC Medical Education Program
Program code: 080-41-11-081
Program type: University-based
State: Pennsylvania
Address: University of Pittsburgh Medical Center,
        Presbyterian South Tower Suite 3880,
        200 Lothrop St, Pittsburgh, PA 15213
Phone: (412) 647-4279
Fax: (412) 647-4788
Percentage of IMGs in the program: 0%
Minimum USMLE Step 1 Score Requirement: No limits set
Minimum USMLE Step 2 Score Requirement: No limits set
Attempts on any step: No limits set
CS required at time of application: Yes including ECFMG certificate
USCE Requirement: None
Cut-Off time since graduation: No limits set
Program offers couple match: Yes
Visas Sponsored or accepted: J1 visa and H1b visa

University of Pennsylvania Dermatology Residency Program

Specialty: Dermatology
Program name: University of Pennsylvania Program
Program code: 080-41-21-080
Program type: University-based
State: Pennsylvania
Address: Hospital of University of Pennsylvania, Department of Dermatology 2 Maloney Building,
3600 Spruce St, Philadelphia, PA 19104
Phone: (215) 662-7883
Fax: (215) 662-7884
Percentage of IMGs in the program: 5%
Minimum USMLE Step 1 Score Requirement: No limits set
Minimum USMLE Step 2 Score Requirement: No limits set
Attempts on any step: No limits set
CS required at time of application: Yes including ECFMG certificate
USCE Requirement: Yes
Cut-Off time since graduation: No limits set
Program offers couple match: Yes
Visas Sponsored or accepted: J1 visa and H1b visa

Thomas Jefferson University Dermatology Residency Program

Specialty: Dermatology
Program name: Thomas Jefferson University Program
Program code: 080-41-11-079
Program type: University-based
State: Pennsylvania
Address: Jefferson Dermatology Associates, Suite 740,
833 Chestnut St, Philadelphia, PA 19107
Phone: (215) 955-4947
Fax: (215) 503-3333
Percentage of IMGs in the program: 8%
Minimum USMLE Step 1 Score Requirement: No limits set
Minimum USMLE Step 2 Score Requirement: No limit set
Attempts on any step: Must pass on first attempt
CS required at time of application: Yes including ECFMG certificate
USCE Requirement: None
Cut-Off time since graduation: No limits set
Program offers couple match: No
Visas Sponsored or accepted: J1 visa and H1b visa

Drexel University College of Medicine/Hahnemann University Hospital Dermatology Residency Program

Specialty: Dermatology
Program name: Drexel University College of Medicine/Hahnemann University Hospital Program
Program code: 080-41-21-077
NRMP Code: 1849080A0
Program type: University-based
State: Pennsylvania
Address: Drexel University College of Medicine, Department of Dermatology MS401,
219 N Broad St, Philadelphia, PA 19107
Phone: (215) 762-5557
Fax: (215) 762-5570
Percentage of IMGs in the program: 0%
Minimum USMLE Step 1 Score Requirement: 220
Minimum USMLE Step 2 Score Requirement: 220
Attempts on any step: No limits set
CS required at time of application: No
USCE Requirement: None
Cut-Off time since graduation: 2 years
Program offers couple match: No

Visas Sponsored or accepted: J1 visa

Penn State Milton S Hershey Medical Center Dermatology Residency Program

Specialty: Dermatology
Program name: Penn State Milton S Hershey Medical Center Program
Program code: 080-41-21-103
State: Pennsylvania
Address: Penn State Milton S Hershey Medical Center, Department of Dermatology,
HU14 500 University Dr, Hershey, PA 17033
Phone: (717) 531-8307   Ext: 3
Fax: (717) 531-6516
Percentage of IMGs in the program: 0%
Minimum USMLE Step 1 Score Requirement: No limits set
Minimum USMLE Step 2 Score Requirement: No limits set
Attempts on any step: No limits set
CS required at time of application: Yes including ECFMG certificate
USCE Requirement: None
Cut-Off time since graduation: No limits set
Program offers couple match: No
Visas Sponsored or accepted: J1 visa

Geisinger Health System Dermatology Residency Program

Specialty: Dermatology
Program name: Geisinger Health System Program
Program code: 080-41-12-076
NRMP Code: 1608080A0
Program type: Community-based university affiliated hospital
State: Pennsylvania
Address: Geisinger Medical Center, Department of Dermatology,
           115 Woodbine Lane, Danville, PA 17822-5206
Phone: (570) 271-8074
Fax: (570) 271-5940
Percentage of IMGs in the program: 0%
Minimum USMLE Step 1 Score Requirement: 210
Minimum USMLE Step 2 Score Requirement: 210
Attempts on any step: No limits set
CS required at time of application: No
USCE Requirement: None
Cut-Off time since graduation: No limits set
Program offers couple match: Yes
Visas Sponsored or accepted: J1 visa

Rhode Island

Brown University Dermatology Residency Program

Specialty: Dermatology
Program name: Brown University Program
Program code: 080-43-21-122
NRMP Code: 1677080A0
Program type: University-based
State: Rhode Island
Address: Rhode Island Hospital/Brown, APC-10, 593 Eddy St, Providence, RI 02903
Phone: (401) 444-7139
Fax: (401) 444-7105
Percentage of IMGs in the program: 0%
Minimum USMLE Step 1 Score Requirement: No limits set
Minimum USMLE Step 2 Score Requirement: No limits set
Attempts on any step: Must pass on first attempt
CS required at time of application: Yes including ECFMG certificate
USCE Requirement: None
Cut-Off time since graduation: No limits set

Program offers couple match: Yes
Visas Sponsored or accepted: J1 visa and H1b
visa

Roger Williams Medical Center Dermatology Residency Program

Specialty: Dermatology
Program name: Roger Williams Medical Center
Program
Program code: 080-43-21-083
State: Rhode Island
Address: Roger Williams Medical Center,
Dermatology & Skin Surgery,
       50 Maude St, Providence, RI 02908
Phone: (401) 456-2521
Fax: (401) 456-6449
Percentage of IMGs in the program: 10%
Minimum USMLE Step 1 Score Requirement:
No limits set
Minimum USMLE Step 2 Score Requirement:
No limits set
Attempts on any step: No limits set
CS required at time of application: No
USCE Requirement: None
Cut-Off time since graduation: No limits set
Program offers couple match: Yes
Visas Sponsored or accepted: J1 visa

South Carolina

Medical University of South Carolina Dermatology Residency Program

Specialty: Dermatology
Program name: Medical University of South Carolina Program
Program code: 080-45-21-099
Program type: University-based
State: South Carolina
Address: Medical University of South Carolina, MSC 578 11th Floor,
        135 Rutledge Ave, Charleston, SC 29425-2215
Phone: (843) 792-9784
Fax: (843) 792-9804
Percentage of IMGs in the program: 0%
Minimum USMLE Step 1 Score Requirement: No limits set
Minimum USMLE Step 2 Score Requirement: No limits set
Attempts on any step: No limits set
CS required at time of application: No
USCE Requirement: Yes

Cut-Off time since graduation: No limits set
Program offers couple match: Yes
Visas Sponsored or accepted: No visa

Tennessee

Vanderbilt University Dermatology Residency Program

Specialty: Dermatology
Program name: Vanderbilt University Program
Program code: 080-47-21-098
Program type: University-based
State: Tennessee
Address: Vanderbilt University Medical Center, One Hundred Oaks Suite 26300,
        719 Thompson Ln, Nashville, TN 37204-3609
Phone: (615) 322-0845
Fax: (615) 343-3947
Percentage of IMGs in the program: 0%
Minimum USMLE Step 1 Score Requirement: No limits set
Minimum USMLE Step 2 Score Requirement: No limits set

Attempts on any step: Must pass on first attempt
CS required at time of application: No
USCE Requirement: Yes
Cut-Off time since graduation: No limits set
Program offers couple match: Yes
Visas Sponsored or accepted: No visa

University of Tennessee Dermatology Residency Program

Specialty: Dermatology
Program name: University of Tennessee Program
Program code: 080-47-21-084
Program type: University-based
State: Tennessee
Address: University of Tennessee Medical Center, Suite H314,
        956 Court Ave, Memphis, TN 38163
Phone: (901) 448-6605
Fax: (901) 448-7836
Percentage of IMGs in the program: 0%
Minimum USMLE Step 1 Score Requirement: 220
Minimum USMLE Step 2 Score Requirement: 220
Attempts on any step: No limits set
CS required at time of application: No
USCE Requirement: None

Cut-Off time since graduation: No limits set
Program offers couple match: Yes
Visas Sponsored or accepted: J1 visa

Texas

Texas A&M College of Medicine-Scott and White Dermatology Residency Program

Specialty: Dermatology
Program name: Texas A&M College of Medicine-Scott and White Program
Program code: 080-48-21-133
NRMP Code: 1725080A0
Program type: Community-based university affiliated hospital
State: Texas
Address: Texas A&M-Scott and White, Northside Clinic,
          409 W Adams, Temple, TX 76501
Phone: (254) 742-7313
Fax: (254) 742-3776
Percentage of IMGs in the program: 0%
Minimum USMLE Step 1 Score Requirement: 220

Minimum USMLE Step 2 Score Requirement:
220
Attempts on any step: Must pass on first attempt
CS required at time of application: Yes including ECFMG certificate
USCE Requirement: None
Cut-Off time since graduation: No limits set
Program offers couple match: Yes
Visas Sponsored or accepted: J1 visa

University of Texas Health Science Center at San Antonio Dermatology Residency Program

Specialty: Dermatology
Program name: University of Texas Health Science Center at San Antonio Program
Program code: 080-48-22-088
State: Texas
Address: University of Texas HSC San Antonio, Medicine/Dermatology MSC 7871, 7703 Floyd Curl Dr, San Antonio, TX 78229-3900
Phone: (210) 567-5673
Fax: (210) 567-4820
Percentage of IMGs in the program: 15%
Minimum USMLE Step 1 Score Requirement:
225

Minimum USMLE Step 2 Score Requirement:
225
Attempts on any step: No limits set
CS required at time of application: No
USCE Requirement: None
Cut-Off time since graduation: No limits set
Program offers couple match: Yes
Visas Sponsored or accepted: J1 visa

Texas Tech University (Lubbock) Dermatology Residency Program

Specialty: Dermatology
Program name: Texas Tech University (Lubbock) Program
Program code: 080-48-21-105
NRMP Code: 2973080A0
Program type: University-based
State: Texas
Address: Texas Tech University HSC Lubbock,
            Department of Dermatology Stop 9400,
            3601 4th St, Lubbock, TX 79430
Phone: (806) 743-2456   Ext: 231
Fax: (806) 743-1105
Percentage of IMGs in the program: 0%
Minimum USMLE Step 1 Score Requirement: No limits set

Minimum USMLE Step 2 Score Requirement: No limits set
Attempts on any step: No limits set
CS required at time of application: Yes including ECFMG certificate
USCE Requirement: None
Cut-Off time since graduation: No limits set
Program offers couple match: Yes
Visas Sponsored or accepted: J1 visa

University of Texas at Houston Dermatology Residency Program

Specialty: Dermatology
Program name: University of Texas at Houston Program
Program code: 080-48-21-100
State: Texas
Address: University of Texas Houston, Department of Dermatology Suite 980, 6655 Travis St, Houston, TX 77030
Phone: (713) 500-8330
Fax: (713) 500-8321
Percentage of IMGs in the program: 8%
Minimum USMLE Step 1 Score Requirement: 230
Minimum USMLE Step 2 Score Requirement: 230

Attempts on any step: Must pass on first attempt
CS required at time of application: Yes including ECFMG certificate
USCE Requirement: None
Cut-Off time since graduation: No limits set
Program offers couple match: Yes
Visas Sponsored or accepted: J1 visa and H1b visa

Baylor College of Medicine Dermatology Residency Program

Specialty: Dermatology
Program name: Baylor College of Medicine Program
Program code: 080-48-21-087
State: Texas
Address: Baylor College of Medicine, Department of Dermatology Suite E6200,
            1977 Butler Blvd, Houston, TX 77030
Phone: (713) 798-7620
Fax: (713) 798-6923
Percentage of IMGs in the program: 0%
Minimum USMLE Step 1 Score Requirement: No limits set
Minimum USMLE Step 2 Score Requirement: No limits set
Attempts on any step: No limits set
CS required at time of application: No

USCE Requirement: None
Cut-Off time since graduation: No limits set
Program offers couple match: Yes
Visas Sponsored or accepted: J1 visa

University of Texas Medical Branch Hospitals Dermatology Residency Program

Specialty: Dermatology
Program name: University of Texas Medical Branch Hospitals Program
Program code: 080-48-11-086
State: Texas
Address: University of Texas Med Branch Hospitals, Department of Dermatology,
301 University Blvd, Galveston, TX 77555-0783
Phone: (409) 772-1911
Fax: (409) 772-1943
Percentage of IMGs in the program: 0%
Minimum USMLE Step 1 Score Requirement: No limits set
Minimum USMLE Step 2 Score Requirement: No limits set
Attempts on any step: No limits set
CS required at time of application: Yes including ECFMG certificate
USCE Requirement: None
Cut-Off time since graduation: No limits set

Program offers couple match: Yes
Visas Sponsored or accepted: J1 visa and H1b visa

University of Texas Southwestern Medical School Dermatology Residency Program

Specialty: Dermatology
Program name: University of Texas Southwestern Medical School Program
Program code: 080-48-21-085
NRMP Code: 2835080A0
Program type: University-based
State: Texas
Address: University of Texas Southwestern Medical Center, Department of Dermatology, 5323 Harry Hines Blvd, Dallas, TX 75390
Phone: (214) 633-1858
Fax: (214) 648-5556
Percentage of IMGs in the program: 0%
Minimum USMLE Step 1 Score Requirement: 230
Minimum USMLE Step 2 Score Requirement: 230
Attempts on any step: Must pass on first attempt
CS required at time of application: No
USCE Requirement: None

Cut-Off time since graduation: No limits set
Program offers couple match: Yes
Visas Sponsored or accepted: J1 visa

Baylor University Medical Center Dermatology Residency Program

Specialty: Dermatology
Program name: Baylor University Medical Center Program
Program code 080-48-13-142:
Program type: University-based
State: Texas
Address: Texas Dermatology Associates, Suite 145,

 3900 Junius St, Dallas, TX 75246
Phone: (972) 386-7546   Ext: 280
Fax: (972) 715-1460
Percentage of IMGs in the program: 0%
Minimum USMLE Step 1 Score Requirement: 220
Minimum USMLE Step 2 Score Requirement: 220
Attempts on any step: No limits set
CS required at time of application: No
USCE Requirement: None
Cut-Off time since graduation: No limits set
Program offers couple match: Yes
Visas Sponsored or accepted: J1 visa

University of Texas Southwestern Medical School (Austin) Dermatology Residency Program

Specialty: Dermatology
Program name: University of Texas Southwestern Medical School (Austin) Program
Program code: 080-48-12-140
NRMP Code: 2835080A1
Program type: Community-based university affiliated hospital
State: Texas
Address: University of Texas Southwestern-Austin,

Dermatology Program Suite C2 470,
601 E 15th St, Austin, TX 78701

Phone: (512) 324-7997
Fax: (512) 324-7969
Percentage of IMGs in the program: 15%
Minimum USMLE Step 1 Score Requirement: 230
Minimum USMLE Step 2 Score Requirement: 230
Attempts on any step: Must pass on first attempt
CS required at time of application: No
USCE Requirement: None
Cut-Off time since graduation: 5 years
Program offers couple match: Yes
Visas Sponsored or accepted: J1 visa

Utah

University of Utah Dermatology Residency Program

Specialty: Dermatology
Program name: University of Utah Program
Program code: 080-49-21-112
Program type: University-based
State: Utah
Address: University of Utah Medical Center, Room 4A330 SOM,
    30 N 1900 E, Salt Lake City, UT 84132
Phone: (801) 581-5509
Fax: (801) 581-6484
Percentage of IMGs in the program: 10%
Minimum USMLE Step 1 Score Requirement: No limits set
Minimum USMLE Step 2 Score Requirement: No limits set
Attempts on any step: No limits set
CS required at time of application: Yes including ECFMG certificate
USCE Requirement: None
Cut-Off time since graduation: No limits set
Program offers couple match: Yes

Visas Sponsored or accepted: J1 visa

Vermont

University of Vermont/Fletcher Allen Health Care Dermatology Residency Program

Specialty: Dermatology
Program name: University of Vermont/Fletcher Allen Health Care Program
Program code: 080-50-13-129
State: Vermont
Address: University of Vermont FAHC,
             FAHC MCHV Campus MS: 250SM1,
             111 Colchester Ave, Burlington, VT 05401
Phone: (802) 847-8770
Fax: (802) 847-8038
Percentage of IMGs in the program: 0%
Minimum USMLE Step 1 Score Requirement: No limits set
Minimum USMLE Step 2 Score Requirement: No limits set
Attempts on any step: No limits set

CS required at time of application: Yes
including ECFMG certificate
USCE Requirement: Yes
Cut-Off time since graduation: 2 years
Program offers couple match: Yes
Visas Sponsored or accepted: J1 visa

Virginia

Virginia Commonwealth University Health System Dermatology Residency Program

Specialty: Dermatology
Program name: Virginia Commonwealth University Health System Program
Program code: 080-51-21-090
NRMP Code: 1743080A0
Program type: University-based
State: Virginia
Address: VCU Medical Center, PO Box 980164, 401 N 11th St, Richmond, VA 23298-0164
Phone: (804) 628-3139
Fax: (804) 827-1909

Percentage of IMGs in the program: 20%
Minimum USMLE Step 1 Score Requirement: 220
Minimum USMLE Step 2 Score Requirement: 220
Attempts on any step: No limits set
CS required at time of application: Yes including ECFMG certificate
USCE Requirement: None
Cut-Off time since graduation: No limits set
Program offers couple match: Yes
Visas Sponsored or accepted: J1 visa

Eastern Virginia Medical School Dermatology Residency Program

Specialty: Dermatology
Program name: Eastern Virginia Medical School Program
Program code: 080-51-21-130
State: Virginia
Address: Eastern Virginia Medical School, Department of Dermatology Suite 200, 721 Fairfax Ave, Norfolk, VA 23507
Phone: (757) 446-0593
Fax: (757) 446-6000
Percentage of IMGs in the program: 0%
Minimum USMLE Step 1 Score Requirement: No limits set

Minimum USMLE Step 2 Score Requirement:
No limits set
Attempts on any step: Must pass on first attempt
CS required at time of application: No
USCE Requirement: Yes 1 month
Cut-Off time since graduation: 2 years
Program offers couple match: Yes
Visas Sponsored or accepted: No visa

University of Virginia Dermatology Residency Program

Specialty: Dermatology
Program name: University of Virginia Program
Program code: 080-51-11-089
NRMP Code: 1737080A0
Program type: University-based
State: Virginia
Address: University of Virginia Health System, Department of Dermatology Box 800718,
1221 Lee St, Charlottesville, VA 22908
Phone: (434) 924-5115
Fax: (434) 924-5936
Percentage of IMGs in the program: 0%
Minimum USMLE Step 1 Score Requirement:
No limits set
Minimum USMLE Step 2 Score Requirement:
No limits set

Attempts on any step: Must pass on first attempt including CS exam
CS required at time of application: Yes including ECFMG certificate
USCE Requirement: None
Cut-Off time since graduation: No limits set
Program offers couple match: Yes
Visas Sponsored or accepted: J1 visa

Washington

University of Washington Dermatology Residency Program

Specialty: Dermatology
Program name: University of Washington Program
Program code: 080-54-31-091
NRMP Code: 1918080A0
Program type: University-based
State: Washington
Address: University of Washington School of Medicine, Box 356524 BB1353,
1959 NE Pacific St, Seattle, WA 98195-6524

Phone: (206) 685-6120
Fax: (206) 543-2489
Percentage of IMGs in the program: 10%
Minimum USMLE Step 1 Score Requirement: No limits set
Minimum USMLE Step 2 Score Requirement: No limits set
Attempts on any step: Must pass on first attempt
CS required at time of application: Yes including ECFMG certificate
USCE Requirement: None
Cut-Off time since graduation: No limits set
Program offers couple match: Yes
Visas Sponsored or accepted: J1 visa and H1b

West Virginia

West Virginia University Dermatology Residency Program

Specialty: Dermatology
Program name: West Virginia University Program
Program code: 080-55-11-092
Program type: University-based

State: West Virginia
Address: West Virginia University Hospitals, PO Box 9158,
　　　　One Medical Center Dr, Morgantown, WV 26506-9158
Phone: (304) 293-9110
Fax: (304) 293-3724
Percentage of IMGs in the program: 0%
Minimum USMLE Step 1 Score Requirement: No limits set
Minimum USMLE Step 2 Score Requirement: No limits set
Attempts on any step: No limits set
CS required at time of application: No
USCE Requirement: None
Cut-Off time since graduation: No limits set
Program offers couple match: Yes
Visas Sponsored or accepted: J1 visa

Wisconsin

Medical College of Wisconsin Affiliated Hospitals Dermatology Residency Program

Specialty: Dermatology

Program name: Medical College of Wisconsin Affiliated Hospitals Program
Program code: 080-56-21-095
State: Wisconsin
Address: Medical College of Wisconsin, Department of Dermatology,
          9200 W Wisconsin Ave, Milwaukee, WI 53226
Phone: (414) 955-3106
Fax: (414) 955-6221
Percentage of IMGs in the program: 8%
Minimum USMLE Step 1 Score Requirement: No limits set
Minimum USMLE Step 2 Score Requirement: No limits set
Attempts on any step: No limits set
CS required at time of application: No
USCE Requirement: None
Cut-Off time since graduation: No limits set
Program offers couple match: Yes
Visas Sponsored or accepted: J1 visa

Marshfield Clinic-St Joseph's Hospital Dermatology Residency Program

Specialty: Dermatology
Program name: Marshfield Clinic-St Joseph's Hospital Program
Program code: 080-56-22-131

NRMP Code: 1780080A1
Program type: Community-based university affiliated hospital
State: Wisconsin
Address: Marshfield Clinic, Dermatology Program,

1000 N Oak Ave, Marshfield, WI 54449
Phone: (715) 389-4151
Fax: (715) 389-4141
Percentage of IMGs in the program: 15%
Minimum USMLE Step 1 Score Requirement: 220
Minimum USMLE Step 2 Score Requirement: 220
Attempts on any step: Must pass on first attempt including CS exam
CS required at time of application: Yes including ECFMG certificate
USCE Requirement: None
Cut-Off time since graduation: 5 years
Program offers couple match: Yes
Visas Sponsored or accepted: J1 visa and H1b visa

University of Wisconsin Dermatology Residency Program

Specialty: Dermatology
Program name: University of Wisconsin Program

Program code: 080-56-21-093
NRMP Code: 1779080A0
Program type: University-based
State: Wisconsin
Address: University of Wisconsin Hospital and
Clinics, Department of Dermatology,
        1 S Park St, Madison, WI 53715
Phone: (608) 287-2658
Fax: (608) 287-2676
Percentage of IMGs in the program: 20%
Minimum USMLE Step 1 Score Requirement:
220
Minimum USMLE Step 2 Score Requirement:
220
Attempts on any step: No limits set
CS required at time of application: Yes
including ECFMG certificate
USCE Requirement: None
Cut-Off time since graduation: No limits set
Program offers couple match: Yes
Visas Sponsored or accepted: J1 visa

I wish you good luck.

Thank you for buying our book.

Please, Please and Please take a minute to review our book on Amazon.

**Match A Doc
Residency Guide**

www.matchadoc.com